The Perils of Sleep Apnea—An Undiagnosed Epidemic

The Perils of Sleep Apnea—An Undiagnosed Epidemic

✦

A Layman's Perspective

Burton Abrams

iUniverse, Inc.

New York Lincoln Shanghai

The Perils of Sleep Apnea—An Undiagnosed Epidemic
A Layman's Perspective

iUniverse books may be ordered through booksellers or by contacting:

iUniverse
2021 Pine Lake Road, Suite 100
Lincoln, NE 68512
www.iuniverse.com
1-800-Authors (1-800-288-4677)

ISBN: 978-0-595-43262-2 (pbk)
ISBN: 978-0-595-87603-7 (ebk)

Printed in the United States of America

This book is dedicated to the memory of my grandfather Max Satinsky, who died in 1946 of a heart attack in his sleep. Sleep apnea was probably the cause.

Contents

Introduction

Shortly after my sleep apnea was diagnosed, I was seated on an airplane flight next to a well-dressed man working assiduously on his laptop computer. Unbridled curiosity drew my eyes as far sideways as possible to view what was on his screen. It looked to me like a picture of the human heart. Having recently contended with my own heart arrhythmia, I found the opportunity to strike up a conversation with him. After I asked about the picture on his screen, he told me that he was an electrophysiologist, which is the cardiology subspecialty dealing with heart rhythm. (Other cardiologists call them the rhythm boys.) And I was seated next to him. What a coincidence!

I steered our conversation to sleep apnea and its impact on cardiac arrhythmia. He referred to sleep apnea as an undiagnosed epidemic. I have kept his words in mind long enough to use them in the title for this book.

Since that conversation, my own research in medical literature has shown me what his words referred to. Published estimates of the percentage of adults in the U.S. with sleep apnea ranging from mild to severe are as high as 20%. That sounds like an epidemic to me! Estimates of the percentage of sleep apneacs (a term that I coined to mean persons with sleep apnea) who have been diagnosed with it are about 5% of those who have it. So my electrophysiologist seat neighbor was right—an undiagnosed epidemic!

But what's the big deal? There are many conditions, athlete's foot for example, which are very common and have a very low percentage of medical diagnosis. Well, the big deal is that sleep apnea has many known serious, even life-threatening, consequences. Those consequences are discussed in this book, including some that are not widely known.

I analogize sleep to the third leg that supports the stool of good health. The other two legs are proper diet and exercise. These two have received much attention, while good sleep has received far too little attention. Yet, without all three legs in good shape, the stool of health may collapse. Furthermore, the three legs are interdependent. Apneacs have been shown to have a less beneficial cardiac response to exercise than others do. And excess weight, from poor diet and/or insufficient exercise, makes the occurrence of sleep apnea more likely.

◆   ◆   ◆

The term apnea derives from Greek and means lack of air. Sleep apnea refers to repeated episodes during sleep in which breathing ceases, each episode lasting for many seconds at a time. If breathing is just greatly reduced rather than stopped entirely, that is termed hypopnea.

Sleep apnea is caused most commonly by an anatomical obstruction in the airway that makes it close up when the muscles relax during sleep. That type of sleep apnea is termed obstructive sleep apnea. The lack of breathing and lack of oxygen in an episode of sleep apnea can be far more severe than one could willingly induce by holding one's breath. The reduction of oxygen, and the accompanying increase of carbon dioxide, in the blood send a signal to the brain's autonomic system that usually jolts the apneac to contract the muscles that open the airway, until the muscles relax again and the cycle is repeated. The apneac usually is not awake during these repeated episodes. But the quality of his sleep is disturbed.

The less common form of sleep apnea is termed central sleep apnea, in which the brain center that controls breathing malfunctions. Some people exhibit a combination of obstructive sleep apnea and central sleep apnea. This book concentrates on obstructive sleep apnea as it affects adults.

◆   ◆   ◆

Three facts about obstructive sleep apnea are recognized by every doctor that I have spoken with: it is very common, it can have very serious consequences, and it is woefully underdiagnosed. Once I gain agreement from a doctor on these three points, I next ask why every adult general physical exam does not include screening for sleep apnea. I have yet to receive a satisfactory answer to that question. I consider the underdiagnosis of sleep apnea to be a major failure of modern medical practice.

Until medical screening for sleep apnea is done as commonly as sphygmomanometer testing for high blood pressure, we the medical laity who are concerned about maintaining our good health are left to our own resources to do our own screening. The first chapter of this book, and some of the second chapter, tell you what to do. They convey the most important information in this book because they let you know how to protect yourself and your loved ones. Much of the rest of this book tells you more about known scientific information about sleep apnea and my hypothesized extensions to that information, all written in layman's language. I have also included a chapter that describes my own sleep apnea experience, and how I came to learn all the information that I present to the readers of this book.

1

The Telltale Signs

In the summer of 2006, my wife and I enjoyed a cruise along the coast of Alaska. Every night aboard ship, there was live entertainment. One of the entertainers was a stand-up comedian who was very funny. He had all of us laughing heartily, including me. Then he reached one part of his routine that I could not laugh at. He described how his brother-in-law would fall asleep in a lounge chair at family get-togethers and snore, then stop breathing, and then restart with a loud snort. The family joked that he might be having a heart attack. The rest of the audience continued laughing.

What the comedian's brother-in-law was displaying are telltale signs of obstructive sleep apnea. And a heart attack, or myocardial infarction, really is a possible outcome of such apneic episodes. To me, and to most people who share my understanding of sleep apnea, snoring is no laughing matter. It is unfortunate that snoring has been depicted in a comedic vein. From Chaucer's "The Canterbury Tales" to Sheridan's play "The Rivals" to the Three Stooges, the strange sounds that people make when snoring have been used for comedy. My kids thought my snoring was funny, and they would tease me about it. But the comedic presentation of snoring has desensitized us to the seriousness of its implications.

◆　　◆　　◆

Snoring is a telltale sign of sleep apnea. Although most people who snore do not have sleep apnea, most people with obstructive sleep apnea are snorers. The key difference is that the apneacs produce a loud snort or gasp that follows a period of no breathing, and no snoring, that lasts for many seconds. When these apneic episodes recur at least five times per hour of sleep, the snorer is displaying the clinical sign of obstructive sleep apnea. They can occur as many as 100 times in an hour in cases of severe sleep apnea.

Most of the time these episodes do not awaken the sleeper to the point of consciousness. The quality of his sleep is disturbed, and the autonomic activity of his brain gets his breathing restarted, but the sleeper usually does not realize that his breathing has been interrupted or that his sleep has been disturbed.

Because the sleeper is unaware of his sleep behavior, the awareness of these telltale signs by his sleeping partner is very important. Whereas the snorer's spouse may be awakened annoyed and disgruntled by the noise of the snoring, medically termed snoring spouse syndrome, it is important that she (or he) use that opportunity to listen for periods of no breathing by which apnea is defined. That telltale sign is better noticed by the sleeping partner than by the sleeper.

I know of a bachelor who has checked his own sleep for these telltale signs by keeping a cassette tape recorder going by his bedside to play back later when he is awake. Listening to eight hours of tape for the sounds of someone sleeping can be pretty tedious, even more tedious than watching paint dry. Furthermore, for the results to be most reliable, several nights should be recorded and checked because the degree of sleep apnea can vary a lot from night to night. I admire this guy's persistence in checking himself for this important health issue.

◆   ◆   ◆

Sometimes a severe apneic episode can awaken the sleeper, although he usually doesn't realize what caused his arousal. What he does realize is that he has the urge to go to the bathroom, an urge that is usually suppressed and controlled while he remains asleep. So another telltale sign can be frequent trips to the bathroom that interrupt sleep.

◆   ◆   ◆

Because sleep is so disturbed and incomplete, a common consequence of sleep apnea is excessive sleepiness at inopportune times during waking hours. This is another telltale sign. A former friend of mine told me how he would often nod off to sleep uncontrollably while sitting at the breakfast table, and then awaken to find his face in his cereal bowl. Other friends of his confirmed to me that he would often doze off while they were out to dinner together. I urged him to pursue the possibility of sleep apnea with his doctor, but he was in denial. I deeply regret that I was not more persistent, because he died from a massive stroke several months later. As described in more detail later in this book, stroke is a common consequence of long-term sleep apnea. While I hate to lose a friend, I would much rather lose a friend by being a nag than lose a friend in this manner. Friends should not let friends ignore sleep apnea.

If it occurs while driving, the effect of uncontrollable sleepiness can threaten life and limb not only of the apneac, but also of passengers in his car or others on the road. Sleep apnea has been recognized as the underlying cause of many traffic accidents. As a safety measure, some European countries have begun requiring that an applicant pass a sleep apnea test before being granted a license for long distance trucking.

◆   ◆   ◆

Another telltale sign may be frequently awakening with a headache. Even beyond that, some headache researchers suspect that sleep apnea may be associated with other headache conditions such as migraine.

◆   ◆   ◆

I have found that an immediate consequence of sleep apnea can be a gout attack that develops while sleeping, which is most commonly the way in which a gout attack begins. Thus, I classify overnight gout attacks as a telltale sign of sleep apnea. This connection is one that I and others have observed when our long-term recurrent gout attacks ceased after the resolution of our sleep apnea. It is a connection not yet recognized by most medical practitioners, even though gout has been associated in medical literature with other causes of oxygen reduction in the body such as moving to a much higher elevation, emphysema, and sickle cell disease. There are reasons for gout other than sleep apnea, and most apneacs do not get gout attacks. But when gout occurs, sleep apnea should be suspected. I devote a major portion of another chapter of this book to the gout/sleep apnea connection, with a description of the physiological reason for it.

◆   ◆   ◆

It may be helpful to be aware that sleep apnea is most common in individuals with certain predisposing characteristics. Family genetics is one predisposing factor. Males are more likely to have sleep apnea than premenopausal females, but after menopause the prevalence in females rises significantly even if hormone replacement therapy is used. Certain physical characteristics such as a deviated septum, or a very thick neck (over 17 inches in circumference), or a receding chin are associated with sleep apnea. Advancing age is a factor too. Sleep apnea is twice as likely to occur at 65 as it is at 45.

The characteristic with the highest coincidence is excess weight. The likelihood of sleep apnea occurrence increases exponentially with excess weight above the recommended level. In the last forty years, the average weight for both men and women in the U.S. has increased by 25 pounds. It's no wonder that the occurrence of sleep apnea has reached epidemic proportions!

But don't get the impression that only overweight people are apneacs. About 30% of apneacs are not obese. I am not, and never was, overweight, and neither are four of the people that I know who have been diagnosed with sleep apnea.

◆   ◆   ◆

To summarize, telltale signs of sleep apnea are:

- Snoring
- Noticeable periods of cessation of breathing while sleeping lasting many seconds
- Excessive sleepiness during waking hours
- Frequent trips to the bathroom that interrupt sleep
- Headache when awakening
- Gout

Remember how many of us are sleep apneacs, and that the vast majority of us don't know it. Since most doctors do not routinely screen their patients for sleep apnea, each of us must use these telltale signs to screen ourselves and our loved ones. The next issue to address is what to do if sleep apnea is suspected. That is the subject of the next chapter.

2

What to do When Sleep Apnea Is Suspected

The obvious response to the issue addressed in this chapter is to consult your primary care physician with the evidence that you have, and prod him or her to follow up in an effective way. But there are things that you can do on your own to gather more evidence and possibly to overcome the apnea.

◆   ◆   ◆

One thing that you can do for more diagnostic information is test the severity of the oxygen deprivation (hypoxia) that you undergo while sleeping. The episodes of apnea result in less oxygen intake, which results in less oxygen carried through the body in the bloodstream's hemoglobin. It is easy to measure the percentage of oxygen saturation in your hemoglobin throughout your sleep by using the proper type of a device called a pulse oximeter. You can rent such a device from a medical equipment company, even though your health insurance probably won't pay for the rental if it's not prescribed by a doctor. I paid $50 to rent one for a four-day weekend.

A pulse oximeter is an electronic device that simultaneously measures both pulse rate and the percentage of oxygen saturation in the blood. It has a sensor that slips over a finger and illuminates it like ET's finger. The sensor is connected via cable to the rest of the meter. The type of pulse oximeter needed for an overnight test is one that has a paper tape printout on which is recorded the readings taken at intervals of a few minutes. After the sleep period is finished, results can be determined by examining the printout. In addition to your own review of the tape, your doctor should review it as well.

Normal oxygen percentage during waking hours is 96%-98% near sea level. (At high elevations, the rarified air reduces the normal percentage level, for which the body gradually compensates over a few weeks time by increasing the number of red blood cells, so that the total amount of oxygen distributed by the blood meets the body's needs.) The normal reduction at sea level during sleep lowers the percentage to about 92%. If the level drops below 90%, that indicates an hypoxia problem during sleep. People with severe sleep apnea may have their readings dip below 80% many times during the sleep interval. It is helpful to perform these readings for several nights because of the variability of the apnea severity.

Be aware that hypoxia may not be pronounced in some apneacs. Also be aware that hypoxia may result even if there is no apnea. In short, testing for hypoxia is not a definitive test for sleep apnea. But it is a very strong indicator, one that your doctor should be made aware of.

◆   ◆   ◆

In addition to self-diagnosis with a pulse oximeter, there are some things that you can do that are likely to alleviate the apnea. One thing is to be sure that you are not overweight. Overweight people are more likely to have sleep apnea because excess flab forms in their airway tissue as well as elsewhere in their bodies, making the airway more likely to close during the relaxation of sleep. About 70% of sleep apneacs are significantly overweight.

It's also a good idea to restrict your drinking of alcoholic beverages so that you have none for several hours before going to sleep. Alcohol in your system makes sleep apnea more likely to occur more severely.

Don't smoke. How often are we given that warning. Yet sleep apnea is one more reason to avoid smoking. It inflames the airway tissues so they start out even before sleep narrowing the airway so that it is more likely to close during sleep.

Be careful about sleep medications. Certain sleep medications, both over the counter and prescription (eg. sedatives), can induce apnea while sleeping. Some apneacs experience insomnia, which makes them seek to use such medications. Ironically, they may only exacerbate the problem.

Another thing that you can do is adopt what is called position therapy while you are sleeping. In common parlance, that means never allow yourself to sleep on your back because in that position gravity can move the base of your tongue so that it is more likely to close up the airway. An effective means to implement this therapy is to pin a sock to the back of your pajama tops and place a tennis ball in the sock. The idea is that if you ever roll over onto your back, the discomfort of the tennis ball will arouse you enough to turn off your back again. This therapy has been shown to be most effective with people who are not overweight. Elevating your head so that it is at an angle of about 30 degrees above horizontal is helpful too.

I have used position therapy with much success. But, since I don't like to wear pajama tops, I cut two slits in a tennis ball through which I slipped an elastic belt. When I went to bed I buckled the belt around my torso with the ball in the back.

In order to test the effectiveness of this ball-in-the-back method, I rented a tape-printout pulse oximeter to use for several nights in my own bed. With the ball, my lowest reading was 94%. I tested without the ball one night and found several times when my percentage dropped to 87%, even though I tried to sleep lying always on my side.

During subsequent use of my belt and tennis ball method, I found that I would occasionally awaken lying on my back with the ball pushed aside. I upgraded my method to straddle my spine using the belt with two tennis balls. Since then I introduced a second upgrade by replacing the tennis balls by Wiffle™ perforated plastic softballs. Compared to the slitted tennis balls, the Wiffle™ balls are larger, less compressible, lighter weight, come with the slits built into them, and dry faster after washing. The one time that I suffered a gout attack with the balls in place, I awakened to find my neck turned so that my body was lying on its side and my head on its back, my wife was complaining about my excessively loud snoring, and my foot was screaming with the searing pain of gout.

After using the ball method for 18 months, I tried for four weeks sleeping without a net, so to speak, to see if I had trained myself well enough to stay off my back without the balls. It worked—no gout. Then I rented a pulse oximeter again for four nights to see if the numbers were good. They were great!

◆   ◆   ◆

If these self-help approaches do not sufficiently solve your problem, you need to rely on medical practitioners for your therapy. The first step in that process is an interview with a physician who specializes in sleep medicine, usually a pulmonologist. He or she will probably arrange to have you undergo an overnight test in a sleep lab. In the lab a technician will connect sensors to many areas of your body, let you fall asleep in a private room, and remotely monitor your sensors to make sure they are functioning properly while you sleep. You may wonder how you will ever be able to fall asleep with all those sensors on you, but you will. If you wake up and have to use the bathroom, you ring for the technician to quickly disconnect your sensor wires first and reconnect them afterwards. In the morning the technician will awaken you and disengage you from all the sensors.

The sleep lab test is called polysomnography. It measures and records many things about your sleep in addition to apnea. One of its problems is that it is very expensive. My bill for a one-night stand was over $6,000. I was very glad to have only a $20 copay, and that my health insurance company was responsible for the balance.

Because of its expense, diagnosis of the severity of sleep apnea usually is made on the basis of a one-night stand. Polysomnography is called the "gold standard" for the diagnosis of sleep apnea, maybe because it is so expensive. Because of the variability of apnea from night to night, the sensitivity of this test is only about 90%. That means that about 10% of the people who have sleep apnea will not be diagnosed with it by one night of polysomnography. Thus, the "gold standard" is slightly tarnished. There certainly is room for new technology to create a diagnostic procedure that is less expensive and more reliable.

◆   ◆   ◆

Once the diagnosis is completed, a therapeutic approach will be recommended. In those limited cases where there is an anatomical abnormality in the airway, surgery to remove it may be recommended. Examples of such cases may be a deviated septum, or an oversized uvula (the punching bag hanging down at the very back of your mouth.) Surgical approaches have met with limited success, and like all surgical procedures, involve some risk. But once the recovery period is over, when surgery achieves the goal no further action is needed.

Another therapy that is beneficial in some cases is the use while sleeping of a specially fitted oral appliance, much like a football player's mouth guard. The appliance positions the jaw and tongue so that snoring and apnea do not occur as long as it stays in place. For this approach to be of benefit, the mouth must be structured in a certain way. Only some apneacs have the structure for this approach to be useful.

By far, the most effective therapy is the use of a mask while sleeping through which air is provided for breathing with Continuous Positive Airway Pressure (CPAP). The CPAP mask provides air to the nose and mouth whose pressure is slightly elevated above the surrounding air pressure, just enough to keep the airway from closing. The pressurized air is delivered to the mask via a wide hose from a bedside pumping machine. CPAP's proper operation requires that the mask be sealed around the nose and mouth and held in place by straps around the back of the head and neck. Complaints sometimes arise about the air being too dry or that the pressure seal chafes too much. The biggest complaint, though, is that the mask is so intrusive and is easily knocked out of place if the user tilts his head to the side. As a result, many users give up in frustration. Here is another area where there is an opportunity for technological improvement. Even with the current drawbacks, when the apneac uses the CPAP mask every night, it is extremely effective.

In some cases, concentrated oxygen may be delivered by a narrow hose to the nostrils. This may help reduce the hypoxia problem in sleep apnea, but it does little for the problem of disturbed sleep.

◆   ◆   ◆

To summarize, therapies to overcome obstructive sleep apnea are:

- Weight loss
- Sleep position
- Surgery
- Oral appliance
- CPAP mask while sleeping
- Concentrated oxygen supply while sleeping.

The first two you can attempt on your own, but the others require you to work with a doctor.

There is no magic elixir or pill to overcome sleep apnea. Each of the therapies has its complications and difficulties. So is it really worth the effort? That issue is discussed in the next chapter.

3

Why Be Concerned

Reggie White was one of those rare professional athletes whose play was so good and unique that he changed the way the game is played. Others now emulate his style of play. He was recognized posthumously by being inducted into the Pro Football Hall of Fame. In the NFL he played defensive end, first for the Philadelphia Eagles, and then for the Green Bay Packers. He was also a man of the cloth, an ordained minister, respected by many who knew him. Sportswriters liked to refer to him as the Minister of Defense. Reggie White died in 2004 at the age of 43, a few years after his retirement from football. He died in his sleep from severe cardiac arrhythmia, as reported in the news of his death. The news also reported that he had sleep apnea, complicated by pulmonary sarcoidosis. Sarcoidosis is an autoimmune disease that causes inflammation which develops lumps of cells in an organ, very often the lungs, lumps that impede the organ's function. Pulmonary sarcoidosis is known to cause ventricular tachycardia, a serious heart arrhythmia which is often fatal. In Reggie's case, neither his athleticism nor his faith could save him from an early death.

An article in the November 10, 2005, issue of the highly regarded New England Journal of Medicine provides some statistics about the perils of sleep apnea. While the article focuses primarily on the connection of sleep apnea to stroke and high blood pressure, it provides some other statistics which to me are the most telling. The authors found that over a period of 3½ years, as compared with people of the same age and sex without sleep apnea, people with untreated sleep apnea have a risk of dying from all causes that is 2 to 3 times higher, depending on the severity of the sleep apnea. If you want the gist of why be concerned about sleep apnea, you don't have to read any further. That's it, in a nutshell.

Maybe you're more concerned about suffering a long debilitating illness than you are about dying. Sleep apnea has many consequences that are debilitating in addition to life threatening. The list is discussed below.

Cardiovascular Diseases

That New England Journal article gives further statistics about the high prevalence of stroke and high blood pressure in patients with long-term sleep apnea. Stroke was found to have the same risk factor as dying over the 3½ year period tested. Furthermore, over 60% of stroke patients were found to have obstructive sleep apnea. High blood pressure that does not respond well to the usual treatments is especially associated with sleep apnea. Fatal heart attacks as well as strokes have both been reported elsewhere to be almost three times more prevalent in apneacs than in nonapneacs. Three times more prevalent! And that's for fatal heart attacks. It's even higher for nonfatal heart attacks.

There are many other cardiovascular diseases whose high association with sleep apnea has been published in medical journals. They include atherosclerosis (plaque deposits in arteries), heart failure, and heart arrhythmias, including atrial fibrillation and ventricular arrhythmia. These cardiovascular diseases make up one of the two groups of diseases most commonly associated with long-term sleep apnea.

In my case, my atrial fibrillation arrhythmia stopped a while after my sleep apnea was resolved. Whereas the cessation of my gout was immediate, the cessation of my atrial fibrillation took more than six months to complete.

It is known that apneacs are subject to sudden death from cardiac causes mostly while sleeping, as happened with Reggie White. Those people without sleep apnea who die suddenly from cardiac causes usually die during waking hours.

◆   ◆   ◆

Neurological Conditions

The second area most commonly associated with long-term sleep apnea is neurological. Foremost in this area are the effects of sleep deprivation, which include grogginess, poor attention span, diminution of mental acuity, clinical depression, and periods of excessive sleepiness. As mentioned previously, the excessive sleepiness is known to lead to traffic accidents by apneacs dozing off at the wheel.

There can be personality changes as well, the type that we can all associate with lack of sleep. These plus impaired memory and decreased executive function can reduce a person's job performance. That plus the inability to stay awake can even cause loss of a job.

The medical community has recently realized that former U.S. President Taft suffered from obvious and debilitating sleep apnea that impaired his job function when he was president. That was in the early part of the twentieth century, and sleep apnea would not be recognized as a medical problem until about fifty years later. When he was president, Taft was severely obese, and he suffered from gout. His journals and his aide's journals record how he frequently fell asleep in the middle of important meetings. When Taft later became Chief Justice of the Supreme Court, he had lost 60-70 pounds, and there is no record of any more inopportune sleeping spells. The complete story is posted at www.apneos.com. That website also provides one of the best descriptions of sleep apnea that I have found.

Some apneacs find that they frequently wake up with a morning headache. That was not one of the symptoms that I experienced.

One of the symptoms that I did experience was occasional periods of severe dizzy spells, periods lasting about five minutes. One time I was coming out of a supermarket when one of those spells caused me to topple to the ground along with my shopping cart. Another time, I had to pull over while driving to wait until the spell passed. After having me tested for all the usual suspects, my neurologist concluded that these dizzy spells were caused by sleep apnea. That was the first time that any doctor mentioned to me the possibility of my sleep apnea. I regret that I didn't follow-up on his conclusion, but I was just grateful to learn that it wasn't anything "serious". At that time I was as ignorant about the dangers of sleep apnea as most people still are. The dizzy spells continued until my sleep apnea was resolved two years later, and then the dizzy spells never recurred.

An additional neurological condition that has been reported to be associated with sleep apnea, but not often mentioned, is Alzheimer's disease. In fact, the two conditions have been shown to be associated with the same genetic variant—APOE epsilon 4.

◆   ◆   ◆

Metabolic Diseases

The primary metabolic diseases known to be associated with sleep apnea are adult-onset diabetes and kidney disease. One study found that 33% of adult-onset diabetics were apneacs. A collection of diseases which often occur together and are known to be associated with sleep apnea is termed the metabolic syndrome. The metabolic syndrome includes diabetes, bad cholesterol and triglyceride numbers, atherosclerosis, high blood pressure, and gout.

◆   ◆   ◆

Autoimmune Diseases

An autoimmune disease is one in which the body's immune system, designed to seek and destroy invading microbes, attacks its own organs. Those diseases whose association with sleep apnea has been published in medical literature include: Hashimoto thyroiditis; amyotropic lateral sclerosis (ALS), commonly called Lou Gehrig's disease; and myasthenia gravis. Investigation of the association of autoimmune diseases with sleep apnea has not received much attention in medical literature. But there is one paper that has found sarcoidosis to be associated with sleep apnea in several more cases than just Reggie White.

◆   ◆   ◆

Gout

As I mentioned previously, I have found that gout attacks are a consequence of sleep apnea. Gout is an extremely painful and inflammatory rheumatic disease whose attacks usually develop while a person is asleep. It is caused by the deposition in a joint of crystals of monosodium urate (MSU). These MSU crystals precipitate from the solution of uric acid in the blood when the solution becomes too concentrated. Uric acid is a natural waste product from the cells' metabolic processes. It is removed from the blood stream and chemically processed by action of the kidneys and of naturally occurring intestinal bacteria. At the time that their blood is tested, most people with gout show uric acid levels in the normal range, indicating that their body's rate of removal of uric acid is keeping up with its rate of production at that time. The best indication, but more difficult to obtain, would be testing the blood during the period of sleep.

In contradistinction to most of the other diseases listed whose association is with long-term sleep apnea, I believe that a gout attack is an immediate result of serious apneic events that significantly elevate the uric acid level and diminish its solubility in the blood during sleep. As such, it is an immediate warning of sleep apnea with a pain so intense that it cannot be ignored.

My primary care physician has begun screening his gout patients for sleep apnea. He has found a large percentage of them to have sleep apnea that was previously undiagnosed. I wish that he could find the motivation to take some time from his busy practice to publish his results.

◆   ◆   ◆

Association or Causality

It is important to establish whether sleep apnea causes any of this long litany of serious diseases, or whether they are associated because of some other root cause. I contend that there is strong reason to believe that sleep apnea is the cause for most of them.

The usual scientific approach to test a causality hypothesis is to introduce the causal agent under controlled conditions where that is the only variable between two otherwise identical groups, and then see if the suspected resultant appears only in the group with the causal agent. No medical researchers are going to purposely induce sleep apnea to see what develops.

Another test for causality is to remove the causal agent whence it is present and see if the suspected resultant disappears, or is at least mitigated. Medical literature has shown that to be the case for diabetes, where resolving sleep apnea in many patients reduced their levels of hemoglobin A1c, which is the "gold standard" marker for diabetes. Other researchers have found that resolving sleep apnea in patients with atherosclerosis reduced the frequency of new serious cardiovascular events such as heart failure. Resolving sleep apnea also has been found to improve high blood pressure. This is important information, not only as evidence for causality, but also as encouragement for apneacs that resolving their sleep apnea can improve their health problems. In other words, resolving sleep apnea is not only preventative, but also curative.

Other evidence for causality is generated when we can identify a causal mechanism that leads from sleep apnea to the resulting diseases. That is the subject of the next chapter.

4

How Sleep Apnea Can Cause So Many Serious Diseases

In this chapter, I will present my hypotheses about how sleep apnea can cause so many serious diseases. I derived all these descriptions by forming connections from my reading of published articles in medical journals. After realizing the connections, I then published these hypotheses in medical journals. Almost all of these diseases result from the repeated apneic episodes of hypoxia, which is the reduction of oxygen in the body.

It is important to note that hypoxia may not be the only cause of these diseases in apneacs. In fact, some apneacs do not exhibit hypoxia. Another causal factor may be the elevated levels of catecholamine hormones (eg. adrenaline) known to be present in apneacs. But my focus in this chapter is on the intermittent hypoxia that so many apneacs undergo every night.

◆   ◆   ◆

Gout

In the late 1980s, pulmonologists were searching for a convenient, reliable way to determine if their critical care patients were receiving enough oxygen. They found that the amount of uric acid in the blood (serum uric acid) and even in the urine (urinary uric acid) could provide the information that they sought.

Pulmonary journal literature from that time and later describes how hypoxia causes the body's cells to begin a process of disintegration, called catabolism, which would lead to cell death if continued long enough. In that process, the adenosine triphosphate (ATP), the chemical component of a cell's protoplasm that stores and supplies its energy, undergoes a series of chemical transitions that culminates in the cell's generation of excess uric acid. Furthermore, when the process reaches that final stage, it is irreversible. That means if the hypoxia in sleep apnea were to be stopped suddenly because the apneac were to start breathing again, it would be too late. The uric acid would not go back up the chemical chain towards ATP. It would remain as uric acid to be removed from the cell and carried away by the blood stream. The uric acid generated as the result of hypoxia is in excess of the amount produced by the cells' normal metabolic processes. More and more is fed into the blood stream with each apneic episode, taxing the kidneys' ability to dispose of it fast enough.

A second result of hypoxia is an imbalance in the blood between oxygen and carbon dioxide, an imbalance tilted toward extra carbon dioxide. Carbon dioxide in solution forms a weak acid, carbonic acid, which is present in all soda pop because of the aeration with carbon dioxide. The imbalance of carbon dioxide over oxygen makes the blood more acidic (lower pH), a condition termed acidosis. The body's control mechanisms act to maintain a very narrow range of pH in the blood (7.35 to 7.45). So more carbonic acid means some blood acid will be discarded, uric acid in particular. The way it's discarded is by the formation of the solid crystalline compound monosodium urate (MSU), which is deposited in the body's connective tissues, or as uric acid kidney stones, which develop in about 40% of gout sufferers.

That's the physiological connection of sleep apnea with gout. The apnea causes hypoxia, which causes acidosis along with excess serum uric acid, which causes MSU precipitation. When MSU lodges in a joint, it causes an attack of gout. When MSU is formed, even if it is not in a joint, it can produce other bad consequences.

◆   ◆   ◆

Autoimmune Diseases

In the fall of 2003, researchers at the University of Massachusetts published a paper that describes one of the reactions of the body's immune
system to MSU. It activates dendritic cells (the immune system's scouts)
which are designed to pick up identifying molecular components of invading microbes and present them to activated T-cells (the immune system's
microbe killers), which also were found to arise as a result of MSU. These
researchers viewed uric acid as a cry for help to the immune system from
dying cells. But the immune system would certainly be greatly overtaxed if
it had to respond to every upward fluctuation of uric acid. There has to be
a threshold to be exceeded for the response to be triggered. These researchers found that the precipitation of MSU is the threshold. When uric acid
was elevated to any point below that level, there was no such immune system response.

Uric acid often is regarded as beneficial in the body. It is an antioxidant
that scavenges for free radicals to protect body tissues from harmful chemical reactions with them. Elevated levels of uric acid have been shown to
reduce the symptoms of multiple sclerosis. It has an anti-inflammatory
effect in a particular type of arthritis. However, some researchers have
shown that elevated uric acid levels may promote kidney disease and high
blood pressure, so the reviews on uric acid are mixed.

On the other hand, MSU gets uniformly bad reviews. It has a pro-
inflammatory effect in the same type of arthritis for which uric acid is anti-
inflammatory. I view the uric acid—MSU dichotomy as a case of too
much of a good thing gone bad. And when MSU from hypoxia activates
the immune system microbe fighters when there are no invading microbes
to fight, that could be really bad.

If that were a rare event, the body could probably take it in stride. But
what if that process is repeated multiple times every night for years, as it
would be with long-term sleep apnea? Each time the immune system's
dendritic cells are up-regulated to pick up identifying molecular compo-

nents of invading microbes, some of them invariably pick up the body's own molecular components and pass them on to killer T-cells. There is a police force in the immune system (mainly in the thymus gland and the bone marrow) which scans these cells for the body's molecular components to destroy them. But no police force is 100% efficient. A small percentage of these cells survive with each episode to do their damage somewhere in the body. There is a strong consensus among immunologists that the repeated up-regulation of such an immune response over a long period of time is crucial for the development of autoimmune disease.

More data are needed to determine if known autoimmune diseases, other than those few listed previously, have a high coincidence with sleep apnea. Even more importantly, studies need to be conducted to see if resolving sleep apnea leads to deceleration, halt, or even reversal of autoimmune disease progress. It is interesting to note that some ophthalmologists have reported that allopurinol, which is a drug commonly used for treating gout because it suppresses the production of uric acid and MSU, has produced extremely beneficial results in the treatment of autoimmune uveitis.

Based on my description of the causal relationship of both autoimmune diseases and gout to sleep apnea, one might expect that there would be a high coincidence of gout and autoimmune diseases. In fact, the only published reports of such coincidences show the opposite to be true. Both rheumatoid arthritis and lupus, which are autoimmune diseases usually treated by rheumatologists, have been reported to have extremely low coincidence with gout. Gout is an autoinflammatory, but not autoimmune, disease whose inflammation is self-limiting. The body's inflammatory reaction to gout is to gradually coat the MSU crystals in the joint, which acts to hide the crystals from sensing by further inflammatory reactants. It may be that gout is a reaction to MSU which some human body's have the capacity to use as a protective mechanism against autoimmune development, somewhat analogous to some individuals having sickle cell disease as a protective mechanism against the more devastating effects of malaria.

◆   ◆   ◆

Diabetes

Juvenile diabetes has been known for a long time to be autoimmune, and I am not suggesting that it is associated with sleep apnea. But adult-onset diabetes is known to be strongly associated with sleep apnea. In recent years, several medical journal papers have been published showing that adult-onset diabetes is also autoimmune in many patients. Data are needed to determine if patients with autoimmune adult-onset diabetes are hypoxic apneacs. In any case, since it is already known that resolving sleep apnea improves diabetes in many patients, the resolution of possible sleep apnea always should be pursued in people with adult-onset diabetes.

◆   ◆   ◆

Cardiovascular Diseases

Atherosclerosis is known to be an inflammatory disease in which plaque is deposited on the interior walls of arteries, which constricts the flow of blood. Medical researchers have tried in vain to find a type of bacteria or virus that causes the body to react with that inflammation. Other research-ers have sought to show that the oxidative stress from sleep apnea was the cause of the inflammation, but their study ended up refuting that hypoth-esis. What has been found is that blood flow is improved in apneacs with atherosclerosis by the use of allopurinol (the gout drug), which is probably an indication that the inflammation was subsiding. This is a piece of evi-dence showing that MSU may be an inflammatory agent that can cause the inflammation of atherosclerosis, and that suppressing the generation of MSU allows the atherosclerosis to subside.

The inflammation of atherosclerosis, which in combination with diabe-tes and gout is one of the metabolic syndrome diseases, is marked by high levels of C-reactive protein in the blood. One study has shown that mea-sured levels of C-reactive protein increase with the severity of sleep apnea.

In addition, a known consequence of sleep apnea is systemic inflammation.

Stroke and hypertension are also known to have a strong association with sleep apnea. The mechanism for that association may be the hypercoagulability (elevated tendency of the blood to clot) that is known to occur in sleep apneacs. There is some evidence that the hypercoagulability may be a manifestation of autoimmunity.

In people with severe and prolonged sleep apnea, the right side of the heart is subjected to pressure from the lungs, which can result in a severe form of congestive heart failure.

◆   ◆   ◆

Alzheimer's Disease

Alzheimer's disease has been hypothesized to be an autoimmune disease in which self-antibodies that are aimed at nerve tissue manage to enter the brain by infiltrating the blood-brain barrier. This connection may explain the reason for the noted strong association of sleep apnea with Alzheimer's disease. The neural self-antibodies may develop from repeated chronic MSU production and T-cell immune response as a result of long-term sleep apnea.

◆   ◆   ◆

Cancer

I have found no published data showing an association of sleep apnea with any type of cancer. Probably that's because no one has looked for any association. But there is a plausible connection that could stimulate such investigations.

There is increasing realization that cancer develops as the result of long-term chronic tissue injury. In some cases it may be long-term exposure to toxic waste, or to cigarette smoke. For stomach cancer, it's long-term exposure to helicobacter pylori bacteria. In cervical cancer, it's long-term exposure to the human papilloma virus.

A person with long-term sleep apnea experiences chronic tissue injury caused by the chronic intermittent episodes of hypoxia. Furthermore, many cancer tumors out of necessity develop a metabolism that acts without oxygen (hypoxic), because they grow so quickly that the blood vessels to supply them can't grow fast enough to keep up. These cancer tumors thrive in hypoxic conditions.

Certain types of cancers are known to be highly associated with obesity. Since sleep apnea is so prevalent with obesity, these types need to be studied for association with sleep apnea. They include: colon, prostate, gall bladder, kidney, esophageal, endometrial, and postmenopausal breast cancers. In fact, all conditions known to have high association with obesity need to be re-examined for their association with sleep apnea.

5

My Personal Experience with Sleep Apnea

Atrial fibrillation (Afib) is a commonly occurring type of cardiac arrhythmia that is known to be a consequence of sleep apnea. Its greatest danger results because its uneven heartbeat disrupts the smooth flow of blood through the heart, allowing the blood to form small pools in which the flow rate is much lower. When blood flow rate slows, the blood is more prone to coagulate (clot). Furthermore, if sleep apnea is involved, the coagulability of the blood is increased. The greatest danger of a prolonged period of atrial fibrillation is that a clot will form in the heart that will break off and be carried by the blood to a location where it gets stuck and then greatly or totally impedes blood flow there. If the clot gets stuck in a blood vessel to the brain, it causes a stroke.

◆　　　◆　　　◆

In the Hospital

That's what happened to me. I had a twenty-hour long period of Afib, which I could judge by sensations in my chest and by feeling the irregularity of my pulse. I knew enough about the danger of a prolonged period of Afib from my cardiologist. He had told me if it continued for 24 hours, I should go to a hospital emergency room to be given intravenous heparin, an anticlotting agent. But when my Afib stopped after 20 hours, I assumed it was safe to forget about the hospital trip. I was wrong.

The next day I became aphasic (couldn't speak), the result of a ministroke called a TIA (transient ischemic attack). I remember being able to formulate thoughts, but I couldn't speak them at my business meeting. My business associates were astute enough to call 911. So I got a ride to the hospital ER in a rescue squad ambulance instead of in my own car.

In the ER, I was assigned to a neurologist who followed the course of my TIA and my aphasia, which had begun to recede after a few hours. By the next morning, I could tell that I had regained almost all of my speech ability. My neurologist came in to my hospital room to see me. I already knew that he had a humorless personality. He asked me, "How's your speech?" I decided to see if I could get him to smile, so I responded, "I'm working on a new one. Tell me what you think." Then I started to recite Lincoln's Gettysburg Address. He refused to smile. I could see that his jaw muscles were clenched to prevent him from smiling. When I finished he said, "I guess you're okay." Then he turned and left. I never saw him again. I had demonstrated to him, and to myself, that all my faculties were restored.

The electrophysiologist assigned to my case was the one who questioned me about sleep apnea, for which I will always be grateful. Fortunately, it was at a time when my wife was present. He first asked me if I ever find that I am excessively sleepy during the day. I told him that I hadn't noticed that. Then he asked if I snore. Before I could answer with a begrudging "Yes," my wife responded with a passionate and animated description of my snoring. He then turned his questioning to her, ignoring me as if I were a piece of the furniture. He next asked if she ever noticed whether I stopped breathing in my sleep. She replied that I did, and that it worried her. That was news to me!

My electrophysiologist arranged for me to have a consultation with a pulmonologist, who had me tested overnight with a pulse oximeter. My blood saturation level dipped down below 80%, well below the 90% threshold level for hypoxia. I was recommended to have further, more extensive testing as an outpatient in the hospital's sleep lab. But to me, the problem was clear, and worrisome.

I remained in the hospital for five days. That was the amount of time required for my dosage of coumadin™ (aka warfarin), an orally administered anticoagulant, to reach the titration level required for it to be effective, but not too high to be seriously dangerous. After all, this is the stuff in rat poison that causes the nasty critters to bleed to death internally. After the first day, I was up and about, walking the halls and stairs, starting to go stir crazy. On the fourth day I was scheduled for a lab test. An orderly showed up with a wheelchair to take me to the lab. I invited him to sit in the chair while I pushed him, following his directions to get to the lab. But he refused. We compromised by walking together to the lab, both pushing the empty chair.

On the fifth day, I was released with a prescription for coumadin™ at a dosage of 5.5 mg per day. I also had an appointment with the pulmonologist to begin a sleep study.

◆   ◆   ◆

In the Sleep Lab

At the sleep lab I was attached to many types of sensors all over my head and body to monitor many things overnight, including sleep apnea. I found out in that test that my blood oxygen saturation level had dipped as low as 88%. It was still below the 90% target, but I wondered why it was so much higher than the 80% measured in the hospital.

In my investigation of sleep apnea, I learned that an effective remedy for some people (usually people who are not overweight) is to avoid sleeping on one's back, since in that position the airway is more likely to become closed. It just so happened that when I went to the sleep lab I was engaged in a bout with sciatica that was more painful when I slept on my back, so I tried not to sleep that way. Previously in the hospital, however, I didn't have the sciatica pain, and I purposely slept on my back to avoid disturbing my IV drip. While I was in the hospital I had a gout attack. I subsequently learned that gout sufferers are more likely to have an attack in the hospital than at home. I now know why.

As a result of that investigation, I adopted the balls-in-the-back method to make sure that I never sleep on my back. That method has worked well for me for 3 ½ years so far, even though I weaned myself from the balls after the first 18 months.

◆   ◆   ◆

After My Resolution of Sleep Apnea

Two things became apparent to me within a month or so after my sleep apnea was resolved. I had not experienced any of the sporadic intense dizzy spells. And I no longer was subjected to attacks of gout, attacks which I had suffered every few weeks with varying degrees of severity for a period of at least fifteen years.

The reason for the gout relief really puzzled me, but I figured that my doctors could explain it. They couldn't. In fact, no doctor that I asked could explain it, except for one. He is a friend of mine, a pediatric nephrologist, very bright, and knowledgeable about many aspects of medicine beyond just his specialty. Within a few seconds after I told him of my observation, he exclaimed, "Of course! Why didn't I think of that!" He then expounded his on-the-spot hypothesis that the excess carbon dioxide in the blood from sleep apnea makes the blood more acidic, which causes uric acid to precipitate from it as monosodium urate. You know from reading Chapter 4 of this book, that is one of the two physiological reasons why gout attacks are caused by sleep apnea.

My doctor friend also told me about how I could learn more by using the Pubmed website, which led to the start of my reading, and writing, medical journal articles. There are more details about that website near the end of this book. All I know is what I read in the papers. When Mark Twain said that, he meant the newspapers. When I say it, I mean the medical journal papers that are accessible through Pubmed.

Other things became apparent over a longer period of time following the resolution of my sleep apnea. One of those things was the gradual decrease in my daily dosage of coumadin™, a dosage that was adjusted regularly based on frequent blood testing that measures coagulation time.

My dosage started at 5.5 mg/day. Over the ensuing six months, it had settled gradually to 3.5 mg/day. I know now that this decrease was the result of my sleep apnea hypercoagulability gradually diminishing. It took a few months to completely subside.

My Afib also took about six months to disappear, even though I was using some pretty strong medication then to control it (amiodarone). Now I am Afib-free, using only a low daily dosage of a time-release beta blocker. My electrophysiologist jokes that beta blockers are so effective for Afib and for controlling high blood pressure, and they are very safe, so they probably should be added to the public water supply like fluorides are.

I was asked recently how I can be sure that I no longer have sleep apnea. I was able to list quickly six answers. I no longer have gout, I no longer have sporadic severe dizzy spells, I no longer have any atrial fibrillation, I no longer have diabetes (which caused me to adopt a low glycemic index diet as well as my sleep regimen), my annual self-checks with a pulse oximeter provide verification, and my wife tells me that I no longer snore. Also, I no longer feel the need to take any midday naps, as I used to allow myself to do regularly on weekends. Oh, and my neck size has gone down from 17 ½ to 16 ½, even though my weight hasn't changed. All that happened from training myself to sleep on my side with my head tilted upward. Even though my list of consequences from sleep apnea is somewhat lengthy, I thank God that nothing more serious has developed.

◆　　◆　　◆

My recommendations about Medical Care

Based on my own medical experiences, there are just a few recommendations that I would offer to all thoughtful individuals who are concerned about maintaining their health.

1. Learn as much as you can from reliable sources about good health practices, and specifically about particular ailments that you may be facing.

2. Link yourself up with the best doctors you can find. The practice of medicine is not monolithic. One of my doctors referred to the practice of medicine as more art than science. To aid you in finding the best doctors, try to find a regional compendium of doctors in various specialties showing how many other doctors voted that they would use the doctors listed for treatment of their loved ones or themselves. Don't accept just one doctor's recommendation about another without further checking. Try to find former or current patients and solicit their opinions. Use the first visit to a new doctor to interview her or him.

3. Never blindly entrust your medical care in the hands of your doctors, even though you have carefully selected them. Question your doctors to gain better understanding of their recommendations. Seek second or third opinions for the treatment of serious conditions. Use the knowledge that you have gained to be the ultimate decision maker for your medical care. Your doctor may be the CEO, but you are the Chairman of the Board.

6

How Modern Medical Practice Has Failed Us

For at least the last 100 years, all physicians were taught as part of their medical school training that gout is caused by excessive levels of uric acid. I am sure that the pulmonologists who wrote about hypoxia leading to excess uric acid knew about the potential for gout development. So we have to wonder why they didn't walk down the hall to talk to the rheumatologists, the specialists in gout treatment.

Or … maybe they did! Maybe the rheumatologists they spoke to chose to ignore the information, preferring not to lose their cash cow gout patients. For the past year and a half, I have been writing emails about the connection that I and others have observed about gout and sleep apnea to roughly 200 gout researchers and practitioners worldwide, most of whom are rheumatologists. I expected that some would test the concept to see if it would lead to a new therapy for gout. The response has been underwhelming. Only two dozen have responded with thanks for the information. Only three gave any indication that they would like to pursue the idea. One responded that he already knew about the connection, and he was surprised that others didn't. (He is a nephrologist, not a rheumatologist.) Another was receptive to the concept to the point where he dubbed it the "Abrams Syndrome." None have responded that they think the idea is incorrect. But none have published any medical journal paper that substantiates it, or refutes it. Their papers about gout treatment are all focused on drugs, diet, and alcohol use, but mainly drugs. Oh, and did I mention drugs?

When I first phoned my rheumatologist to tell him of my observations, his initial response was to reply excitedly, "Boy, if we could cure gout by curing sleep apnea, that would be great!" The emotional inflection in his voice was very unusual for him. When I phoned him a few weeks later with further information, his demeanor showed complete lack of interest. I can only speculate why his response was so positive in the first phone call, and so uninterested in the second. He did not indicate that on further reflection, he thought the idea was flawed. Could it be that he and his partners realized how much business they would lose if their gout patients were no longer treated in their practice?

The fact that many gout sufferers could be spared the extreme pain of gout and the risk of toxic side effects from gout suppressing drugs is very important. But it is even more important to use gout as a warning of sleep apnea, whose consequences can be life threatening. And those risk levels recede when the apnea is resolved.

◆   ◆   ◆

Johns Hopkins, one of the most highly regarded medical institutions, publishes an on-line health newsletter called Johns Hopkins Health Alerts, which is available by subscription at no charge. In the issue for the week of Oct. 29—Nov.4, 2006, there was an article by one of their cardiologists titled *The ABCs of Heart Attack Prevention*. Here is the complete list of his recommendations: use low dose aspirin daily, control your blood pressure, lower your cholesterol, watch your diet, exercise daily, don't smoke, make sure your blood sugar is under control. Do you notice what is not on that list? It includes nothing about preventing or overcoming sleep apnea. Ironically, the very next article in that issue was about sleep apnea, reporting that heart attack is three times more prevalent in apneacs than in others. Three times! Furthermore, overcoming sleep apnea by using CPAP puts the prevalence of heart attack back down again. In spite of the large number of medical journal articles about it, this cardiologist, and most other cardiologists that I have spoken to, just haven't gotten the message yet about the enormous effect of sleep apnea on the prevalence and prevention of heart attacks. One cardiologist pointed out to me that it is a subject that is almost never mentioned in cardiology journals. My scan of Pubmed listings verified what he said, at least in American cardiology journals.

The Nov. 5-11, 2006, issue of the same Johns Hopkins publication carried an article titled *Simple Steps to Help you Prevent High Blood Pressure Without Medication*. The recommendations are weight loss, healthy diet, regular exercise, and restricting alcohol usage. Once again, there was no mention of sleep apnea. These lapses highlight the failure of modern medical practice.

◆   ◆   ◆

As I mentioned in the Introduction, whenever I speak to a doctor about sleep apnea, I can get agreement on three points: (1) sleep apnea is very common; (2) sleep apnea can have very serious consequences; (3) sleep apnea is woefully underdiagnosed. See if you don't get the same agreement from your doctor. But when I then ask the next question about why adult physical exams don't include routine screening for sleep apnea, I get a response that is either one of ignorance or one of apathy. The apathetic response is often a shrug or a comment that it is not accepted practice. There is not even enough interest to try home use of a pulse oximeter. The ignorant response is that it would require expensive testing in a sleep lab where the majority of people would test negative, and besides, there aren't enough sleep lab facilities to accommodate everybody.

That response shows that the physician is ignorant of the published short, simple office procedures which can do initial screening very effectively. Procedures that describe morphometrics, body measurements that concentrate on the nose, mouth, and jaw, have been written about in medical literature. But the most telling screening practice that has been published in a medical journal is one that involves asking three questions. (1) Do you snore? (2) Do you find that you have periods of excessive sleepiness during waking hours? (3) Does your sleeping partner ever notice that you have periods of many seconds when you stop breathing in your sleep? The family practice doctors who recommend these three questions found that use of these questions increased by eightfold the number of patients diagnosed with sleep apnea. It was these questions posed to me that began my sleep apnea diagnosis and resolution. A more detailed list of questions is also available, referred to as the Berlin questionnaire.

Every family practice physician should be doing that type of screening. Every internist should be doing it. Every cardiologist should be doing it. Endocrinologists should do it. Rheumatologists should do it Nephrologists should do it. And this list is sure to grow as more information is developed about the consequences of sleep apnea.

◆   ◆   ◆

There is one group of physicians who are closely attuned to the consequences of sleep apnea. They are, of course, the sleep medicine physicians. Their initial training is usually in pulmonology, or sometimes in neurology or psychiatry. They lecture and write about the hazards of sleep apnea. But they are lecturing at their own specialized conferences and writing in their own specialized journals. Their culpability is that they are preaching too often to the choir, and not enough to their medical colleagues in other specialties. They should be shouting from the tallest soap box they can find and stop being so collegial in the face of their colleagues' ignorance and apathy. The reason that the sleep apnea epidemic is so underdiagnosed is the epidemic of ignorance and apathy about it among so many doctors.

◆   ◆   ◆

So what are we to do, we who care about preventing health problems as well as having them well treated when they arise? We are left to our own devices to screen ourselves and our loved ones, and to prod our doctors about proper attention to this issue. I've tried to present in this book information that will help you do those things. You can find much more information by searching for sleep apnea websites. You can search an up-to-date catalog list of what's been published in all peer-reviewed medical journals about this topic, or any medical topic, at the Pubmed website operated by the National Institutes of Health at www.ncbi.nlm.nih.gov/entrez/query.fcgi. Pubmed adds over 100 papers every month about the hazards of sleep apnea and the methods and benefits of overcoming it. Many of the listings include a free abstract, which usually synopsizes very well the information in that article. Some complete articles are accessible on line at no charge, and most of the others are available for a single-article fee from their publishers. The articles that I have found apropos to my studies are referenced in the next section.

Stay informed, and stay well.

References

These are medical journal references, organized by topic as discussed in this book. Several of them are listed under multiple topics.

Sleep Apnea—Epidemiology and Consequences

Brown, LK. 2002. A Waist Is a Terrible Thing to Mind: Central Obesity, the Metabolic Syndrome, and Sleep Apnea Hypopnea Syndrome (editorial). *Chest* 122(3): 774-778.

Gami AS. 2005. Day-night pattern of sudden death in obstructive sleep apnea. *New England Journal of Medicine.* 352(12): 1206-1214.

Silverberg, DS, et al. 2002. Treating Obstructive Sleep Apnea Improves Essential Hypertension and Quality of Life. *American Family Physician* 65(2): 229-236.

Teramoto S, Yamamoto H, Yamaguchi Y, Namba R, Ouchi Y. 2005. Obstructive sleep apnea causes systemic inflammation and metabolic syndrome. *Chest* 127(3): 1074-1075.

White DP. 2006. Sleep Apnea. *Proceedings of the American Thoracic Society* 3(1): 124-128.

Yaggi HK. 2005. Obstructive sleep apnea as a risk factor for stroke and death. *New England Journal of Medicine* 353(19): 2034-2041.

Young T, Peppard PE, Gottlieb DJ. 2001. Epidemiology of obstructive sleep apnea: a population health perspective. *American Journal of Respiratory Critical Care Medicine* 165(9): 1217-1239.

Gout, Uric Acid, and Hypoxia

Abrams, B. 2005. Gout Is an Indicator of Sleep Apnea. *Journal SLEEP* 28(2): 275.

Atdjian M, Fernandez-Madrid F. 1981. Coexistence of chronic tophaceous gout and rheumatoid arthritis. *Journal of Rheumatology* 8(6): 989-992.

Du, X., et al. 2005. Significance of the Changes of Urinary Uric Acid in OSAHS Before and After UPPP. *Lin Chuang Er Bi Hou Ke Za Zhi* 19(18): 826-827.

Garcia, AR., et al. 2006. Blood Uric Acid Levels in Patients with Sleep-Disordered Breathing. *Archivos de Bronconeumologia* 42 (10): 492-500.

Grum, CM. 1992. Cells in Crisis: Cellular Bioenergenics and Inadequate Oxygenation in the Intensive Care Unit. *Chest* 102(2): 329-30.

Hasday, JD, Grum, CM. 1987. Nocturnal Increase of Urinary Uric Acid: Creatine Ratio: a Biological Correlate of Sleep-Associated Hypoxemia. *American Review of Respiratory Diseases* 135: 534-38.

Jefferson JA, et al. 2002. Hyperuricemia, hypertension, and proteinuria associated with high-altitude polycythemia. *American Journal of Kidney-Disease* 39(6): 1135-1142.

Khokhar, N. 1980. Hyperuricemia and Gout in Secondary Polycythemia Due to Chronic Obstructive Pulmonary Disease. *Journal of Rheumatology* 7(1): 114-116.

Khokhar, N. 1982. Gouty Arthritis in Chronic Obstructive Pulmonary Disease. *Archives of Internal Medicine* 142(4): 838.

Khosla P, et al. 2004. Concomitant gout and rheumatoid arthritis—a case report. *Indian Journal of Medical Sciences* 58(8): 349-352.

McKeon, JL., et al. 1990. Urinary Uric Acid with Obstructive Sleep Apnea. *American Review of Respiratory Diseases* 142 (1): 8-13.

Navarra SV, Saavedra SC, Cayco AV. 2001. Renal microtophi in a patient with lupus nephritis and tophaceous gout. *Journal of Clinical Rheumatology* 7(4): 268-272.

Plywaczewski, R., et al. 2005. Hyperuricemia in Males with Obstructive Sleep Apnea (OSA). *Pneumonologia i Alergologia Polska* 73(3): 254-259.

Reynolds MD. 1983. Gout and hyperuricemia associated with sickle-cell anemia. *Seminars in Arthritis and Rheumatism* 12(4): 404-413.

Rose DM, et al. 2006. Transglutaminase 2 limits murine peritoneal acute gout-like inflammation by regulating macrophage clearance of apoptotic neutrophils. *Arthritis and Rheumatism* 52(10): 3363-3371.

Ruiz, G.A., et al. 2006. Blood Uric Acid Levels in Patients with Sleep-Disoriented Breathing. *Archives of Bronconeumonology* 42(10): 492-500.

Saito, H., et al. 2002. Tissue Hypoxia in Sleep Apnea Syndrome as Assessed by Uric Acid and Adenosine. *Chest* 121 (55): 1686-1694.

Sahebjani, H. 1998. Changes in Urinary Uric Acid Excretion in Obstructive Sleep Apnea Before and After Therapy with Nasal Continuous Positive Airway Pressure. *Chest* 113(6): 1604-1608.

Uric Acid and Monosodium Urate

Heinig M, Johnson RJ. 2006. Role of uric acid in hypertension, renal disease, and metabolic syndrome. *Cleveland Clinic Journal of Medicine* 73(12): 1059-1064.

Shi Y, Evans JE, Rock KL. 2003. Molecular identification of a danger signal that alerts the immune system to dying cells. *Nature* 425: 516-521.

Zare F, et al. 2006. Uric acid, a nucleic acid degradation product, down-regulates dsRNA-triggered arthritis. *Journal of Leucocyte Biology* 79(3): 482-488.

Autoimmune Disease

Abrams B. 2005. Long-term sleep apnea as a pathogenic factor for cell-mediated autoimmune disease. *Medical Hypotheses* 65(6): 1024-1027.

Drakesmith H, Chain B, Beverley P. 2000. How can dendritic cells cause autoimmune disease? *Immunology Today* 21(5): 214-217.

Erden S, Cagatay T, Buyukozturk S, Kiyan E, Cuhadaroglu C. 2004. Hashimoto thyroiditis and obstructive sleep apnea syndrome: is there any relation between them? *European Journal of Medical Research* 9(12): 570-572.

Ludewig B, Junt T, Hengartner H, Zinkernagel RM. 2001. Dendritic cells in autoimmune diseases. *Current Opinion in Immunology* 13(6): 657-662.

Mehling A, Beissert S. 2003. Dendritic cells under investigation in autoimmune disease. *Critical Reviews in Biochemistry and Molecular Biology* 38(1): 1-21.

Morel PA, Feili-Harriri M, Coates PT, Thomson AW. 2003. Dendritic cells, T cell tolerance and therapy of adverse immune reactions. *Clinical and Experimental Immunology* 133(1): 1-10.

Poluektov MG. 2004. Sleep apnea in neurological disorders. *Zhurnal Nevrologii Psikhiatrii Imeni S. S. Korsakova* 104(3):4-7.

Pulendran B. 2004. Immune activation: death, danger and dendritic cells. *Current Biology* 14(1): R30-32.

Quera-Salva MA, et al. 1992. Breathing disorders during sleep in myasthenia gravis. *Annals of Neurology* 31(1): 86-92.

Shi Y, Evans JE, Rock KL. 2003. Molecular identification of a danger signal that alerts the immune system to dying cells. *Nature* 425: 516-521.

Tsutsumi Z, Moriwaki Y, Takahashi S, Ka T, Yamamoto T. Oxidized low-density lipoprotein autoantibodies in patients with primary gout: effect of urate lowering therapy. *Clinical Chimical Acta* 339(1-2): 117-122.

Vanderlugt CL, Miller SD. 2002. Epitope spreading in immune-mediated diseases: implications for immunotherapy. *Nature Reviews Immunology* 2(2): 85-95.

Heart Disease and Atherosclerosis

Arter JL, Chi DS, Girish M, Fitzgerald SM, Guha B, Krishnaswamy G. 2004. Obstructive sleep apnea, inflammation, and cardiopulmonary disease. *Frontiers in Bioscience* 9: 2892-2900.

El Solh AA, et al. 2006. Allopurinol improves endothelial function in sleep apnoea: a randomized controlled study. *The European Respiratory Journal* 27(5): 997-1002.

Gami AS. 2005. Day-night pattern of sudden death in obstructive sleep apnea. *New England Journal of Medicine.* 352(12): 1206-1214.

Marin JM, Carizzo SJ, Vincente E, Agusti AG. 2005. Long-term cardiovascular outcomes in men with obstructive sleep apnoea-hypopnoea with or without treatment with continuous positive airway pressure: an observational study. *Lancet* 365(9464): 1046-1053.

Milleron O, et al. 2004. Benefits of obstructive sleep apnea treatment in coronary artery disease: a long-term follow-up study. *European Heart Journal* 25(9): 709-711.

Schafer, H., et al. 2002. Body Fat Distribution, Serum Leptin, and Cardiovascular Risk Factors in Men with Obstructive Sleep Apnea (Clinical Investigations). *Chest* 122(3): 829-839.

Shamsuzzaman AS, Winnicki M, Lanfranchi P, Wolk R, Kara T, Accurso V, Somers VK. 2002. Elevated C-reactive protein in patients with obstructive sleep apnea. *Circulation* 105(21): 2462-2464.

Svatikova A, et al. 2005. Oxidative stress in obstructive sleep apnoea. *European Heart Journal* 26(22): 2435-2439.

Tsutsumi Z, Moriwaki Y, Takahashi S, Ka T, Yamamoto T. Oxidized low-density lipoprotein autoantibodies in patients with primary gout: effect of urate lowering therapy. *Clinical Chimical Acta* 339(1-2): 117-122.

von Kanel R, Dimsdale JE. 2003. Hemostatic alterations in patients with obstructive sleep apnea and the implications for cardiovascular disease. *Chest* 124(5): 1956-1967.

Wolk R, Somers VK. 2003. Cardiovascular consequences of obstructive sleep apnea. *Clinics in Chest Medicine* 24(2): 195-205.

Stroke

Anderson HA, Shacter E. 2004. Natural anticoagulant proteins in the regulation of autoimmunity: potential role of protein S. *Current Pharmaceutical Design* 10(8): 929-937.

Guardiola JJ, Matheson PJ, Clavijo LC, Wilson MA, Fletcher EC. 2001. Hypercoagulability in patients with obstructive sleep apnea. *Sleep Medicine* 2(6): 517-523.

Kahn MJ. 2003. Hypercoagulability as a cause of stroke in adults. *Southern Medical Journal* 6(4): 350-353.

Yaggi HK. 2005. Obstructive sleep apnea as a risk factor for stroke and death. *New England Journal of Medicine* 353(19): 2034-2041.

Diabetes

Babu AR, Herdegen J, Fogelfeld L, Shott S, Mazzone T. 2005. Type 2 diabetes, glycemic control, and continuous positive airway pressure in obstructive sleep apnea. *Archives of Internal Medicine* 165(4): 447-452.

Brooks-Worrell BM, Juneja R, Minokadeh A, Greenbaum CJ, Palmer JP. 1999. Cellular immune responses to human islet proteins in antibody-positive type 2 diabetic patients. *Diabetes* 48(5): 983-988.

Harsch IA, Hahn EG, Konturek PC. 2005. Insulin resistance and other metabolic aspects of the Obstructive Sleep Apnea Syndrome. *Medical Science Monitor* 11(3): RA70-75.

Kawasaki E, et al. 2003. Epitope analysis of GAD65 autoantibodies in Japanese patients with autoimmune diabetes. *Annals of the New York Academy of Sciences* 1005: 440-448.

Palmer JP. 2002. Beta cell rest and recovery—does it bring patients with latent autoimmune diabetes in adults to euglycemia? *Annals of the New York Academy of Sciences* 958: 89-98.

Pickup JC. 2004. Inflammation and activated innate immunity in the pathogenesis of type 2 diabetes. *Diabetes Care.* 27(3): 813-823.

Pietropaolo M, Barinas-Mitchell E, Kuller LH, Trucco M. 2000. Is type 2 diabetes a chronic inflammatory-autoimmune disease? *Diabetes* 49(1): 32-38.

Wilding J. 2006. Diabetes and Sleep Apnoea: a hidden epidemic? *Thorax* 61(11): 928-929.

Alzheimer's Disease

Abrams B. 2005. Long-term sleep apnea as a pathogenic factor for cell-mediated autoimmune disease. *Medical Hypotheses* 65(6): 1024-1027.

D'Andrea MR. 2005. Add Alzheimer's disease to the list of autoimmune diseases. *Medical Hypotheses* 64(3): 458-463.

Gottlieb DJ, et al. 2004. APOE epsilon 4 is associated with obstructive sleep apnea/hypopnea: the Sleep Heart Health Study. *Neurology* 63(4): 664-668.

Hoch CC, et al. 1986. Sleep-disordered breathing in normal and pathological aging. *Journal of Clinical Psychiatry* 47(10): 499-503.

Kadotani H, et al. 2001. Association between apolipoprotein E epsilon 4 and sleep-disordered breathing in adults. *Journal of the American Medical Association.* 286(12): 1447-1448.

Inflammation

Arter JL, Chi DS, Girish M, Fitzgerald SM, Guha B, Krishnaswamy G. 2004. Obstructive sleep apnea, inflammation, and cardiopulmonary disease. *Frontiers in Bioscience* 9: 2892-2900.

Teramoto S, Yamamoto H, Yamaguchi Y, Namba R, Ouchi Y. 2005. Obstructive sleep apnea causes systemic inflammation and metabolic syndrome. *Chest* 127(3): 1074-1075.

Allopurinol

EL Solh AA, et al. 2006. Allopurinol improves endothelial function in sleep apnoea: a randomized controlled study. *The European Respiratory Journal* 27(5): 997-1002.

Grus FH, Augustin AJ, Loeffler K, Lutz J, Pfeiffer N. 2003. Immunological effects of allopurinol in the treatment of experimental autoimmune uveitis (EAU) after onset of the disease. *European Journal of Ophthalmology* 13(2): 185-191.

Namazi MR. 2004. Celtrizine and allopurinol as novel weapons against cellular autoimmune disease. *International Immunopharmacology* 4(3): 349-353.

Tsutsumi Z, Moriwaki Y, Takahashi S, Ka T, Yamamoto T. Oxidized low-density lipoprotein autoantibodies in patients with primary gout: effect of urate lowering therapy. *Clinical Chimical Acta* 339(1-2): 117-122.

Cancer

Abrams B. 2007. Cancer and sleep apnea—the hypoxia connection. *Medical Hypotheses* 68(1): 232.

Beachy PA, Karhadkar SS and Berman DM. 2004. Tissue repair and stem cell renewal in carcinogenesis. *Nature* 432(7015): 324-331.

Rubenstein AH. 2005. Obesity: a modern epidemic. *Transactions of the American Clinical and Climatological Association* 116: 103-111.

Wu XZ. 2006. Hypoxia: A common mechanism of tumorigenesis? *Medical Hypotheses*, 67(5): 1252.

978-0-595-43262-2
0-595-43262-X

www.ingramcontent.com/pod-product-compliance
Lightning Source LLC
Chambersburg PA
CBHW050336290526
45785CB00006B/2522